Erectile

DYSFUNCTION

Signs of Impotence and How to Get
a Healthy Sperm for Pregnancy
Before Getting Married

DR. GEORGE FOSTER

TABLE OF CONTENTS

Introduction

In vast human experience, few endeavors are as profound and exhilarating as the quest to create life. It's a journey woven with dreams, hopes, and aspirations, where every step forward is laden with anticipation and possibility. Yet, for some, this journey may present unexpected hurdles, casting shadows of doubt and frustration along the path. It is to these seekers of parenthood, to those navigating the complexities of fertility and sexual health, that this book extends its guiding light.

Imagine a couple, Jack and Sarah, standing at the threshold of matrimony, their hearts brimming with excitement for the adventures that lie ahead. However, as they delve deeper into their relationship, they encounter an unexpected twist—the daunting specter of impotence. Jack's struggles with erectile dysfunction cast a shadow over their dreams of starting a family, leaving them bewildered and uncertain. Yet, amidst the darkness, a glimmer of hope emerges as they embark on a journey of discovery, uncovering the signs of impotence and charting a course towards healing and wholeness.

Similarly, meet David, a man driven by the fervent desire to embrace fatherhood. His path is strewn with obstacles, chief among them the enigma of sperm health. As he immerses himself in the labyrinth of fertility, David learns of the profound significance of healthy sperm in the intricate dance of conception. With each revelation, he gains newfound clarity and determination, fueling his resolve to cultivate fertile grounds for the seeds of life to flourish.

These narratives, though fictional, reflect the myriad experiences of individuals traversing the landscape of fertility and sexual health. Whether grappling with the physical manifestations of impotence or navigating the intricacies of sperm health, their stories resonate with the universal longing for love, connection, and the fulfillment of parenthood.

In the pages that follow, we embark on a voyage of understanding and empowerment, shedding light on the signs of impotence and illuminating the path to healthy sperm and vibrant fertility. Through storytelling, insightful exploration, and practical guidance, we embark on a journey of transformation—a journey that transcends the confines of biology and touches the very essence of human longing and resilience.

So, dear reader, let us embark together on this odyssey, guided by the beacon of knowledge and the compass of hope, as we navigate the boundless seas of fertility and embark on the timeless quest for parenthood.

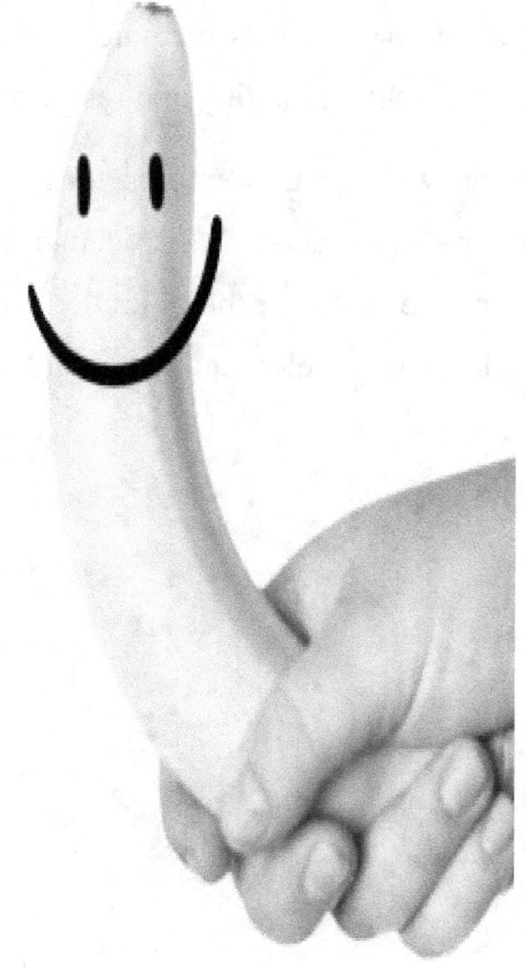

Chapter 1

Understanding Impotence and Breaking Down the Stigma

Impotence, also known as erectile dysfunction (ED), is a condition that affects millions of men worldwide, yet it remains shrouded in stigma and misunderstanding. This article aims to delve into the intricacies of impotence, exploring its causes, symptoms, impacts, and potential treatments. By shedding light on this often-taboo topic, we hope to foster greater understanding and support for those affected by impotence.

Impotence is the term used to describe the persistent inability to obtain or sustain an erection strong enough for sexual activity. Periodically having trouble getting an erection is normal, but repeated problems could point to a health risk. Impotence can affect men of all ages but becomes more common with advancing age.

There are several physiological and psychological causes of impotence. Obesity, diabetes, high blood pressure, heart disease, and hormone abnormalities are common physical causes. Impotence can also result from psychological issues such as interpersonal issues, stress, worry, and despair. Psychological factors such as stress, anxiety, depression, and relationship problems can also contribute to impotence. Additionally, certain lifestyle habits like smoking, excessive alcohol consumption, and drug abuse can increase the risk.

The primary symptom of impotence is the inability to achieve or sustain an erection. Other signs may include reduced sexual desire, premature ejaculation, or delayed ejaculation. It's essential to differentiate between occasional episodes of erectile difficulty and persistent dysfunction lasting for several months, as the latter warrants medical attention.

Beyond its physical manifestations, impotence can profoundly impact mental health and overall well-being. Feelings of inadequacy, embarrassment, and frustration are common among men grappling with impotence. These emotional challenges can strain relationships, lead to social withdrawal, and contribute to the development of anxiety and depression.

Impact on Relationships

Impotence can strain intimate relationships, leading to communication breakdowns and decreased emotional intimacy. Partners may feel rejected or unattractive, exacerbating feelings of insecurity and resentment. Open and honest communication, along with mutual support and understanding, are crucial for navigating these challenges and preserving relationship harmony.

Fortunately, impotence is a highly treatable condition with various options available. Treatment may involve lifestyle modifications such as adopting a healthy diet, regular exercise, and smoking cessation. Medications like Viagra, Cialis, and Levitra are commonly prescribed to improve erectile function. Other approaches include hormone therapy, penile injections, vacuum devices, or surgical implants. Psychological counseling or sex therapy can also be beneficial, particularly for addressing underlying emotional issues.

Breaking the Stigma

One of the biggest barriers to seeking help for impotence is the stigma surrounding the condition. Men may feel ashamed or emasculated, leading them to suffer in silence rather than seek assistance. It's crucial to challenge these societal taboos and promote open discussions about impotence. By normalizing conversations around sexual health and encouraging men to prioritize their well-being, we can empower individuals to seek the support and treatment they deserve.

Impotence is a prevalent yet often misunderstood condition with far-reaching implications for physical and mental health. By fostering greater understanding and empathy, we can break down the stigma associated with impotence and provide vital support to those affected. Through education, advocacy, and access to comprehensive care, we can empower individuals to overcome impotence and reclaim fulfilling, satisfying lives.

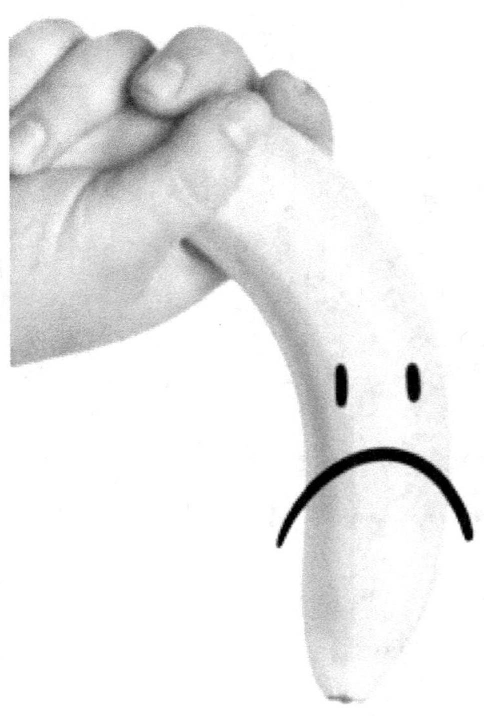

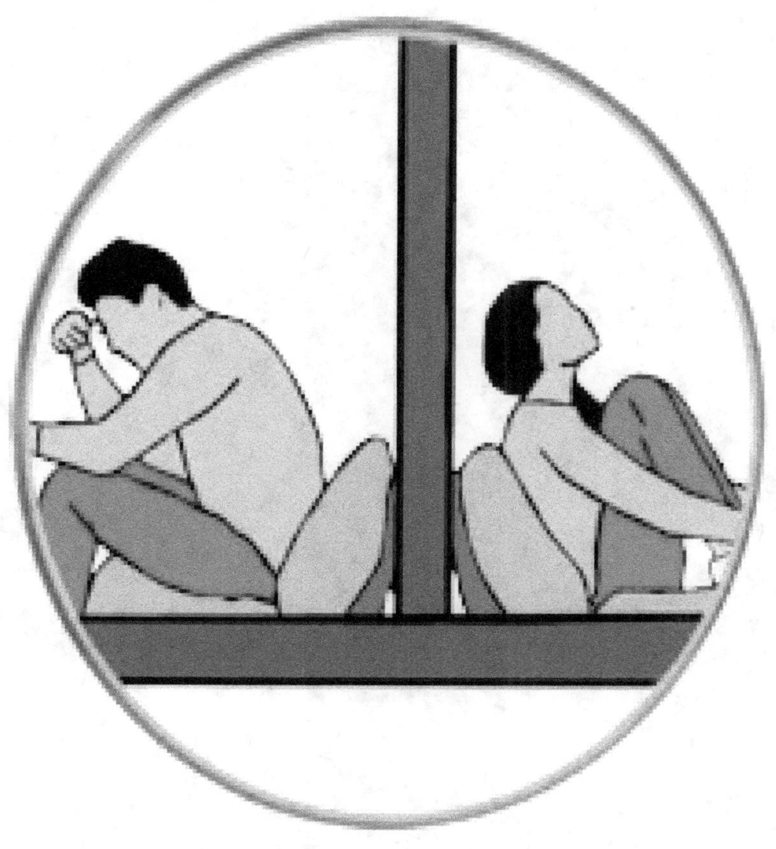

Chapter 2

The Importance of Healthy Sperm for Pregnancy

When it comes to conceiving a child, the health of sperm plays a crucial role. Healthy sperm are essential for successful fertilization and the development of a healthy pregnancy. In this article, we will explore the significance of healthy sperm for pregnancy and discuss factors that can impact sperm health.

Sperm are the male reproductive cells responsible for fertilizing the female egg during conception. For pregnancy to occur, sperm must be able to swim efficiently through the female reproductive tract, penetrate the egg, and deliver their genetic material. Healthy sperm possess certain characteristics that contribute to their ability to perform these functions effectively.

One of the key factors in determining sperm health is sperm count, which refers to the number of sperm present in a semen sample. A healthy sperm count typically ranges from 15 million to 200 million sperm per milliliter of semen. Having an adequate sperm count increases the likelihood of sperm reaching and fertilizing the egg.

In addition to sperm count, sperm motility is another important aspect of sperm health. Motility refers to the ability of sperm to move in a coordinated and purposeful manner. Sperm with high motility are better able to navigate through the female reproductive tract to reach the egg. Poor sperm motility can hinder the fertilization process and reduce the chances of conception.

Sperm morphology, or the size and shape of sperm, also plays a role in fertility. Sperm with abnormal morphology may have difficulty penetrating the egg, leading to decreased fertility. Ideally, a high percentage of sperm in a semen sample should have a normal size and shape to maximize the chances of successful fertilization.

Furthermore, sperm vitality, which refers to the percentage of live sperm in a semen sample, is crucial for fertility. Healthy sperm should have high vitality, indicating that they are capable of fertilizing an egg. Low sperm vitality can significantly reduce the likelihood of conception.

Several factors can influence the health of sperm and affect fertility. Lifestyle factors such as smoking, excessive alcohol consumption, and drug use can impair sperm production and function. Poor diet, obesity, and lack of exercise can also have negative effects on sperm health. Additionally, exposure to environmental toxins, such as pesticides and pollutants, can damage sperm DNA and decrease fertility.

Medical conditions such as genetic disorders, infections, and hormonal imbalances can also impact sperm health. Certain medications, chemotherapy, and radiation therapy can have adverse effects on sperm production and quality. Men need to address any underlying health issues and consult with a healthcare provider if they are experiencing fertility problems.

Fortunately, there are steps men can take to improve sperm health and enhance fertility. Adopting a healthy lifestyle that includes a balanced diet, regular exercise, and avoiding harmful substances can support optimal sperm production and function. Avoiding exposure to environmental toxins and practicing safe sex can also help protect sperm health.

Healthy sperm are essential for pregnancy and the conception of a child. Sperm count, motility, morphology, and vitality all play important roles in fertility. By understanding the factors that influence sperm health and taking proactive steps to support it, men can increase their chances of achieving a successful pregnancy with their partner.

How Infections Affect Sperm Health

Infections can have a significant impact on sperm health, potentially leading to reduced fertility or even infertility in some cases. Various types of infections can affect sperm health, with some directly targeting the reproductive organs or disrupting the body's overall immune function. Here's an overview of the effects of infection on sperm health and the types of infections that can affect it:

Sexually Transmitted Infections (STIs)

STIs are among the most common infections that can affect sperm health. Diseases such as chlamydia, gonorrhea, and genital herpes can cause inflammation and damage to the reproductive organs, including the testes, epididymis, and prostate gland. Inflammation in these organs can impair sperm production, motility, and morphology, leading to decreased fertility. Additionally, some STIs can result in scarring or blockages in the reproductive tract, further hindering the passage of sperm.

Urinary Tract Infections (UTIs)

While UTIs primarily affect the urinary system, they can also impact sperm health if left untreated. UTIs can lead to inflammation and infection in the prostate gland (prostatitis) or seminal vesicles, which are essential for sperm production and transport. Infections in these reproductive organs can disrupt sperm function and decrease fertility.

Urogenital Infections

Infections that affect the urogenital system, such as epididymitis (inflammation of the epididymis) or orchitis (inflammation of the testicles), can have a direct impact on sperm health. These conditions often result from bacterial or viral infections and can cause pain, swelling, and damage to the reproductive organs. In severe cases, urogenital infections may lead to scarring or blockages that impair sperm production and transport.

Systemic Infections

Infections that affect the body's overall immune system can indirectly impact sperm health by disrupting normal physiological processes. Conditions such as HIV/AIDS, tuberculosis, and certain viral infections can weaken the immune system, making individuals more susceptible to reproductive infections or impairing reproductive function directly. Systemic infections can also increase inflammation and oxidative stress throughout the body, which can negatively affect sperm quality and fertility.

Prostate Infections (Prostatitis)

Infections of the prostate gland can cause inflammation and discomfort, leading to pain during ejaculation and reduced sperm quality. Chronic prostatitis may result in long-term damage to the prostate and impair fertility.

Epididymal Infections

The epididymis, a duct located behind the testicles, is responsible for storing and transporting sperm. Infections of the epididymis, known as epididymitis, can disrupt sperm maturation and motility, affecting fertility.

Testicular Infections

Infections of the testicles, such as orchitis, can lead to inflammation and swelling, potentially damaging sperm-producing tissues (seminiferous tubules) and reducing sperm production.

The effects of infection on sperm health can vary depending on factors such as the type and severity of the infection, the duration of exposure, and individual differences in immune response. It's essential for individuals experiencing symptoms of infection, such as pain, swelling, or abnormal discharge in the genital area, to seek medical attention promptly. Early detection and treatment of infections can help prevent complications and minimize the impact on sperm health and fertility.

Infections can have detrimental effects on sperm health by causing inflammation, damage to reproductive organs, and disruptions to normal physiological processes. Sexually transmitted infections, urinary tract infections, urogenital infections, and systemic infections can all impact sperm production, motility, morphology, and overall fertility. Timely diagnosis and treatment of infections are essential for preserving sperm health and optimizing reproductive outcomes.

Chapter 3

How to treat infection affecting sperm Health

Treating infections affecting sperm health typically involves a combination of medical interventions aimed at eliminating the underlying infection, reducing inflammation, and restoring normal reproductive function. The specific treatment approach will depend on the type of infection, its severity, and individual factors such as overall health and medical history. Some common treatment strategies for infections affecting sperm health:

1. **Antibiotic Therapy:** For bacterial infections such as sexually transmitted infections (STIs), urinary tract infections (UTIs), prostatitis, and epididymitis, antibiotic therapy is often the primary treatment. Antibiotics target the

underlying bacterial pathogens responsible for the infection, helping to eliminate the infection and reduce inflammation in the reproductive organs. It's essential to complete the full course of antibiotics as prescribed by a healthcare provider to ensure effective treatment and prevent the recurrence of the infection.

2. **Antiviral or Antifungal Medications:** Infections caused by viruses or fungi, such as genital herpes or candidiasis, may require antiviral or antifungal medications for treatment. These medications work by inhibiting the replication of the virus or fungus, thereby reducing symptoms and preventing the spread of the infection. Antiviral drugs like acyclovir or valacyclovir are commonly used to manage viral infections, while antifungal medications such as fluconazole are effective against fungal infections.

3. **Anti-inflammatory Medications:** Inflammatory conditions affecting the reproductive organs, such as prostatitis or epididymitis, may require anti-inflammatory medications to reduce swelling, pain, and discomfort. Nonsteroidal anti-inflammatory drugs (NSAIDs) like ibuprofen or naproxen can help alleviate symptoms of inflammation and improve overall comfort during treatment. In some cases, corticosteroid medications may be prescribed for more severe or chronic inflammatory conditions.

4. **Pain Management:** Pain associated with infections affecting the reproductive organs, such as testicular pain or pelvic discomfort, may require additional pain management strategies. Over-the-counter pain relievers like acetaminophen or prescription pain medications may be recommended to alleviate pain and improve quality of life during treatment. Heat therapy, such

as warm compresses or sitz baths, can also help relieve discomfort and promote relaxation of the affected tissues.

5. **Supportive Care:** In addition to medical treatment, supportive care measures can help promote healing and recovery from infections affecting sperm health. Adequate rest, hydration, and nutritious diet are essential for supporting the immune system and enhancing overall well-being. Avoiding activities that exacerbate symptoms, such as strenuous exercise or sexual intercourse, may also be recommended until the infection resolves.

6. **Follow-up Care:** After completing the initial course of treatment, follow-up care is important to monitor the effectiveness of treatment and ensure resolution of the infection. Follow-up appointments with a healthcare provider may involve physical exams, laboratory tests, or

imaging studies to assess the status of the infection and reproductive health. Additional treatment or adjustments to the treatment plan may be necessary based on the individual's response to therapy. Overall, early detection and prompt treatment of infections affecting sperm health are essential for minimizing complications and optimizing reproductive outcomes. Individuals experiencing symptoms of infection or fertility issues should seek medical evaluation and appropriate care from a qualified healthcare pro______ ___ treatment and ma___ement, ma_______ ______ eated, res_______ _______ ances of _

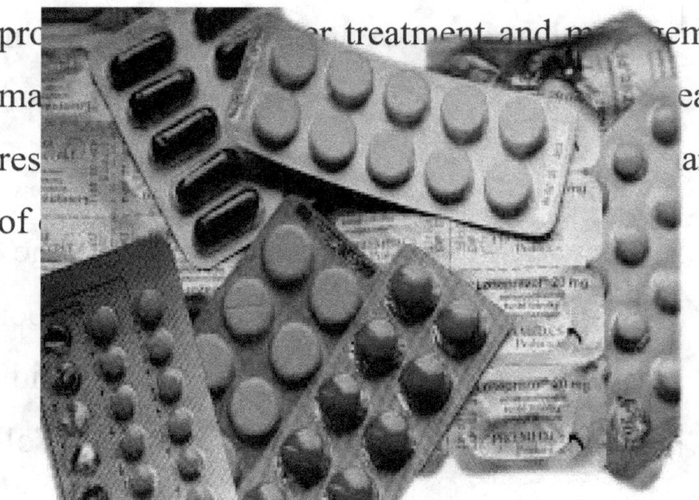

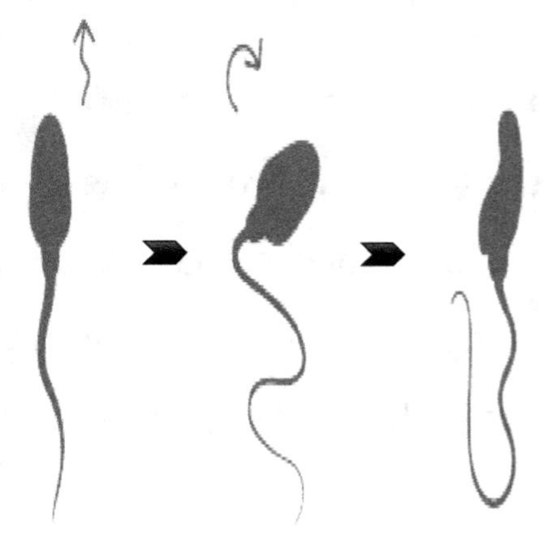

Sperm Morphology and motility
Normal sperm with forward progression
Abnormal motility
Abnormal sperm shape

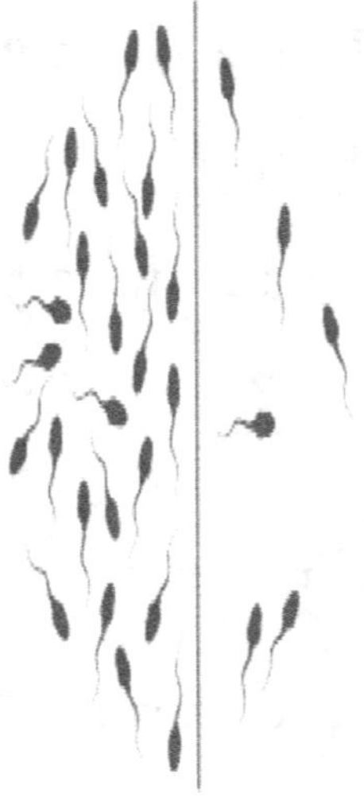

Sperm Count
Normal sperm count
Low sperm count

Chapter 4

Recognizing Signs of Impotence

Erectile dysfunction affects millions of men worldwide. Recognizing the signs of impotence is the first step toward seeking proper diagnosis and treatment.

Difficulty Achieving or Maintaining Erections

One of the primary signs of impotence is difficulty achieving or maintaining erections that are firm enough for sexual intercourse. While occasional erectile difficulties are normal, persistent problems in this area may indicate underlying issues with sexual function.

Reduced Sexual Desire

Another common sign of impotence is a decrease in sexual desire or libido. Men experiencing impotence may find that they have less interest in sexual activity or feel less aroused than usual. This lack of desire can contribute to difficulties with achieving and sustaining erections.

Premature Ejaculation or Delayed Ejaculation

Impotence can also manifest as changes in ejaculatory function. Some men may experience premature ejaculation, where they ejaculate before or shortly after penetration, while others may have delayed ejaculation, where they have difficulty reaching orgasm even with prolonged sexual stimulation.

Anxiety or Stress Related to Sexual Performance

Men with impotence often experience significant anxiety or stress related to their sexual performance. They may worry about their ability to satisfy their partner or feel embarrassed about their erectile difficulties. This psychological distress can further exacerbate the problem and contribute to a vicious cycle of impotence.

Relationship Problems

Impotence can strain intimate relationships, leading to communication breakdowns, resentment, and decreased emotional intimacy. Partners may feel rejected or unattractive, further adding to the stress and pressure surrounding sexual activity.

Underlying Health Conditions

In some cases, impotence may be a sign of underlying health conditions such as cardiovascular disease, diabetes, obesity, high blood pressure, or hormonal imbalances. Men experiencing persistent erectile difficulties should undergo a thorough medical evaluation to identify and address any potential underlying health issues.

Lifestyle Factors

Certain lifestyle factors can also contribute to impotence, including smoking, excessive alcohol consumption, drug abuse, and lack of exercise. Making healthy lifestyle changes, such as quitting smoking, moderating alcohol intake, and maintaining a healthy weight, can improve erectile function and overall sexual health.

Psychological and Emotional Indicators

1. **Anxiety and Stress:** Psychological factors such as anxiety and stress often play a significant role in the development and persistence of impotence. The fear of not being able to perform sexually can create a cycle of anxiety, leading to further difficulties with erections.

2. **Depression and Low Self-Esteem:** Impotence can take a toll on mental health, leading to feelings of depression, low self-esteem, and worthlessness. Individuals may experience a sense of inadequacy or failure, further impacting their confidence and overall well-being.

3. **Relationship Strain:** The emotional impact of impotence can extend to relationships, causing strain and tension between partners. Communication breakdowns, feelings of resentment, and a lack of intimacy may result from the challenges posed by impotence.

When to Seek Medical Help

If you or your partner are experiencing any of the signs and symptoms mentioned above, it's essential to seek medical help promptly. A healthcare provider can conduct a thorough evaluation to determine the underlying cause of impotence and recommend appropriate treatment options.

Treatment for impotence may include lifestyle modifications, such as adopting a healthy diet and exercise regimen, as well as medications like Viagra, Cialis, or Levitra to improve erectile function. In some cases, counseling or sex therapy may be beneficial for addressing psychological factors contributing to impotence.

Overall, recognizing the signs of impotence and seeking timely medical intervention can help restore sexual function and improve the overall quality of life for men and their partners. Don't hesitate to reach out to a healthcare provider if you have concerns about your sexual health or experience persistent erectile difficulties.

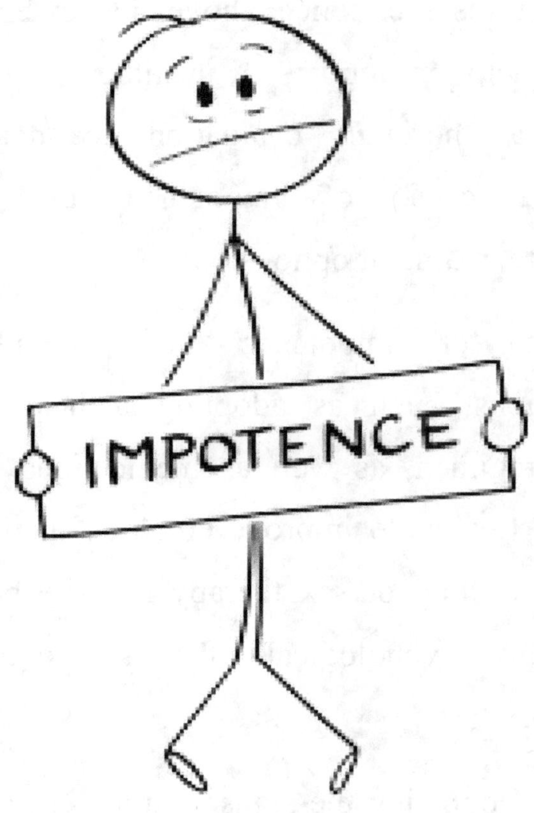
IMPOTENCE

Chapter 4

Optimizing Sperm Health for Fertility

Achieving pregnancy often involves a combination of factors, with sperm health playing a crucial role in the process. Optimizing sperm health is essential for couples trying to conceive, as healthy sperm increase the likelihood of successful fertilization and pregnancy. In this guide, we'll explore various strategies for improving sperm health and enhancing fertility.

Maintain a Healthy Lifestyle

A healthy lifestyle is fundamental for supporting optimal sperm health. This includes following a balanced diet rich in fruits, vegetables, whole grains, lean proteins, and healthy fats. Avoid excessive consumption of processed foods, sugary beverages, and high-fat meals, as they may negatively impact sperm quality. Additionally, regular exercise, adequate sleep, and stress management techniques can contribute to overall well-being and improve sperm health.

Avoid Tobacco, Alcohol, and Drugs

Tobacco smoking, excessive alcohol consumption, and illicit drug use have been linked to decreased sperm quality and fertility. Men who smoke are more likely to have lower sperm counts, reduced sperm motility, and higher rates of sperm abnormalities. Similarly, heavy alcohol consumption and drug abuse can impair sperm production, disrupt hormone levels, and contribute to erectile dysfunction. Quitting smoking, moderating alcohol intake, and avoiding recreational drugs can help improve sperm health and fertility.

Maintain a Healthy Weight

Obesity has been associated with decreased sperm quality and fertility in men. Excess body weight can disrupt hormonal balance, increase oxidative stress, and contribute to conditions such as insulin resistance and metabolic syndrome, all of which can negatively impact sperm production and function. Achieving and maintaining a healthy weight through regular exercise and a nutritious diet can help optimize sperm health and improve fertility.

Practice Safe Sex

Practicing safe sex is important for preventing sexually transmitted infections (STIs) that can damage reproductive organs and impair sperm health. STIs such as chlamydia, gonorrhea, and genital herpes can cause inflammation, scarring, and blockages in the reproductive tract, leading to decreased fertility. Using condoms consistently and correctly during sexual activity can help reduce the risk of STIs and protect sperm health.

Manage Chronic Health Conditions

Chronic health conditions such as diabetes, hypertension, and autoimmune disorders can negatively impact sperm health and fertility. Men with these conditions need to work closely with healthcare providers to manage their health effectively. Proper management of chronic conditions through medication, lifestyle modifications, and regular medical monitoring can help minimize their impact on sperm health and fertility.

Limit Exposure to Environmental Toxins

Exposure to environmental toxins such as pesticides, heavy metals, and industrial chemicals can adversely affect sperm health and fertility. Men who work in industries with potential exposure to harmful substances should take precautions to minimize contact and use protective equipment when necessary. Additionally, adopting environmentally friendly practices at home, such as using natural cleaning products and organic pesticides, can help reduce exposure to toxins and support sperm health.

Consider Supplements and Antioxidants

Some studies suggest that certain supplements and antioxidants may help improve sperm health and fertility. These include vitamins C and E, selenium, zinc, coenzyme Q10, and L-carnitine. However, it's essential to consult with a healthcare provider before starting any supplements, as they may interact with medications or have side effects.

Seek Medical Evaluation and Treatment

If you and your partner have been trying to conceive without success, it's essential to seek medical evaluation and treatment from a fertility specialist. A comprehensive fertility assessment can help identify any underlying issues affecting sperm health and fertility, such as hormonal imbalances, genetic disorders, or structural abnormalities. Depending on the findings, treatment options may include medication, lifestyle modifications, assisted reproductive techniques (ART), or surgery.

Optimizing sperm health is crucial for couples trying to conceive. By adopting a healthy lifestyle, practicing safe sex, managing chronic health conditions, limiting exposure to environmental toxins, considering supplements and antioxidants, and seeking medical evaluation and treatment when needed, men can improve sperm health and enhance fertility. Working together with healthcare providers and adopting proactive measures can increase the chances of achieving a successful pregnancy and fulfilling the dream of parenthood.

Lifestyle Modifications for Enhanced Sperm Quality

Achieving optimal sperm quality is vital for couples trying to conceive, as healthy sperm are essential for successful fertilization and pregnancy. While genetics play a role in sperm health, lifestyle factors also significantly impact sperm quality. By making certain lifestyle modifications, men can improve sperm health and enhance their chances of fathering a child

There lived a man named Mr. Billy. He had always dreamed of starting a family with his beloved wife, Mrs. Lily. However, despite their unwavering love for each other, they faced a challenge on their journey to parenthood - Mr. Billy's struggle with infertility.

Determined to overcome this obstacle, Mr. Billy embarked on a quest to optimize his sperm health and enhance their chances of conceiving a child. At the dawn of 2021, he made a solemn vow to make positive lifestyle modifications that would bring him closer to his dream of fatherhood.

The first step on Mr. Billy's journey was to maintain a healthy weight. He knew that obesity could negatively impact sperm quality, so he resolved to shed the excess pounds that had crept up over the years. With dedication and perseverance, he embraced a balanced diet filled with fruits, vegetables, lean proteins, and whole grains. Gone were the days of unhealthy snacks and sugary treats. Instead, he nourished his body with wholesome foods that fueled his determination to improve his sperm health.

Next, Mr. Billy turned his attention to his habits of indulgence. He bid farewell to his old vices, vowing to limit his alcohol intake and quit smoking for good. With each sip of water in place of alcohol and each breath of fresh air untainted by smoke, he felt a sense of liberation and empowerment.

But Mr. Billy's journey didn't end there. He knew that managing stress was crucial for optimal sperm health. He took up meditation and mindfulness practices, finding solace in the stillness of his mind and the rhythm of his breath. With each moment of tranquility, he felt the weight of worry and anxiety lifting from his shoulders, leaving behind a sense of peace and calm.

As Mr. Billy continued his quest, he embraced the joy of regular exercise. He explored the parks and trails of the town, reveling in the beauty of nature as he jogged, biked, and hiked his way to better health. With each step and stride, he felt his body growing stronger and more resilient, ready to face the challenges of fatherhood.

And finally, Mr. Billy made a solemn promise to himself and Mrs. Lily to practice safe sex. They understood the importance of protecting themselves from sexually transmitted infections that could harm their reproductive health. With love and trust as their guiding principles, they embraced this commitment wholeheartedly.

As the months passed and the seasons changed, Mr. Billy's efforts began to bear fruit. He noticed subtle changes in his body and mind - increased energy, improved mood, and a sense of vitality that he hadn't felt in years. And then, one day, their prayers were answered - Mrs. Lily discovered that she was pregnant.

With tears of joy streaming down their faces, Mr. Billy and Mrs. Lily embraced each other, knowing that their journey to parenthood had finally reached its destination. And as they awaited the arrival of their bundle of joy, they reflected on the power of love, determination, and the transformative impact of lifestyle modifications on their journey to enhanced sperm quality and fertility. For Mr. Billy, 2021 would forever be remembered as the year that he became a father - a testament to the strength of the human spirit and the miracles that await those who dare to dream.

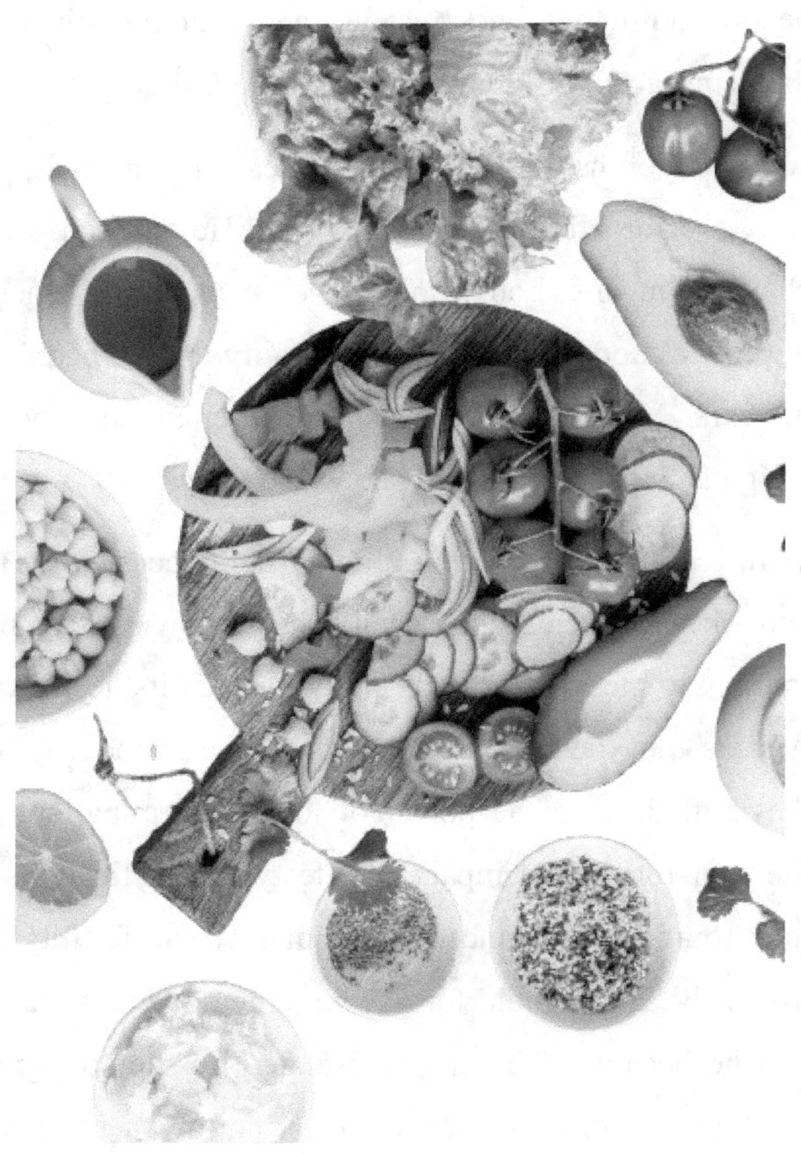

Chapter 5

How to Boost Sperm Count and Motility

Nutritional strategies play a crucial role in enhancing sperm count and motility, which are vital factors for male fertility. Incorporating these nutritional strategies into your diet and lifestyle may help boost sperm count and motility, ultimately improving male fertility

Maintain a Balanced Diet: Consuming a well-rounded diet rich in fruits, vegetables, whole grains, lean proteins, and healthy fats provides essential nutrients necessary for optimal sperm production and function.

Increase Antioxidant Intake: Antioxidants such as vitamins C and E, selenium, and zinc help protect sperm from oxidative stress, which can damage sperm DNA. Foods high in antioxidants include citrus fruits, berries, leafy green vegetables nuts and seed.

Omega-3 Fatty Acids: Incorporating sources of omega-3 fatty acids, such as fatty fish (salmon, mackerel, sardines), flaxseeds, chia seeds, and walnuts, may improve sperm quality by reducing inflammation and enhancing membrane fluidity.

Zinc-Rich Foods: Zinc is crucial for sperm production and testosterone metabolism. Foods rich in zinc include oysters, beef, poultry, dairy products, beans, and nuts. Adequate zinc intake may help increase sperm count and motility.

Folic Acid: Folic acid, also known as vitamin B9, is essential for sperm production and DNA synthesis. Foods high in folic acid include leafy greens, beans, lentils, fortified cereals, and avocado.

Lycopene: Lycopene, a powerful antioxidant found in tomatoes, watermelon, pink grapefruit, and other red or pink fruits and vegetables, has been associated with improved sperm motility.

Avoid Excessive Alcohol: Excessive alcohol consumption can impair sperm production and quality. Limiting alcohol intake or abstaining altogether may help improve sperm health.

Moderate Caffeine Consumption: While moderate caffeine intake is generally considered safe, excessive caffeine consumption may negatively impact sperm quality. Limiting caffeine from sources like energy drinks tea and coffee may be beneficial.

Maintain a Healthy Weight: Obesity has been linked to reduced sperm quality and fertility. Maintaining a healthy weight through a balanced diet and regular exercise may help improve sperm parameters.

Stay Hydrated: Adequate hydration is essential for overall health, including sperm production and motility. Drinking plenty of water throughout the day supports proper bodily functions.

Reduce Exposure to Environmental Toxins: Minimize exposure to environmental toxins such as pesticides, heavy metals, and chemicals, which can negatively affect sperm production and quality.

Consider Supplements: In addition to obtaining nutrients from food, certain supplements like coenzyme Q10, carnitine, and vitamin D may also support sperm health. However, it's essential to consult with a healthcare provider before starting any new supplements.

Incorporating these nutritional strategies into your diet and lifestyle may help boost sperm count and motility, ultimately improving male fertility